2018 Glute
Buyers Guide

MW00927750

Table of Contents

Introduction by Josh Schieffer

First, let me thank you for picking up this book. We are delighted you have decided to find the best in gluten-free. This book has been carefully designed to help you quickly connect with the best gluten-free products, services, and organizations. We host the Annual Gluten-Free Awards; a program that enables the gluten-free community to cast votes for their favorites. This year we had 3,102 people take part in the voting process. The 83,310 individual responses are all rolled up in the following pages.

This year we changed the cover design and added a few new award categories now totaling 60.

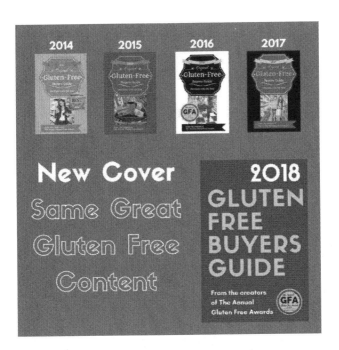

Our Story

The story behind The Gluten Free Awards that very few people know

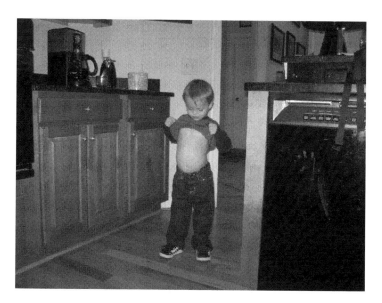

I remember it like it was yesterday when my four-year-old son Jacob, now thirteen, was playing in the kiddie pool with other kids that I assumed were his age based on their height. After asking all the surrounding kids what ages they were, I realized Jacob was significantly smaller than kids his own age. This prompted my wife and I to seek a professional opinion. After consulting with our family physician, she confirmed that Jacob had essentially stopped growing for an entire year without us realizing it. He was referred to Jeff Gordon's Children's Hospital in Charlotte North Carolina to discuss possible growth hormone therapy. The doctors there reviewed Jacob's case and requested a few blood tests based on some suspicions they had.

Our cell phone service at our house was terrible so when the doctor finally called with the blood results, my wife and I ran to the front of the driveway to hear the doctor clearly. With a sporadic signal, we heard "Jacob has celiac disease." We looked at each other as tears ran down my wife's face. We huddled closer to the phone and asked, "what is celiac disease?". After getting a brief description mixed with crappy cell service and happy neighbors waving as they drove by, my wife and I embraced and wept. We were told to maintain his normal diet until we could have an endoscopy and biopsy for further confirmation. Once confirmed our next visit was to a registered dietitian for guidance.

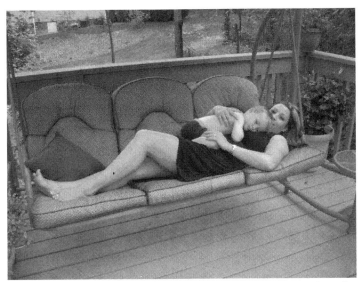

Jayme, my wife, made the appointment and called me with a weird request. "Will you meet me at the dietitian's house for a consultation?". I was confused when she said to go to her house. Jayme then explained that the dietician's daughter had celiac disease too and the best way to show the new lifestyle to patients would be to dive right in. I'll admit, it was a bit uncomfortable at first to be in a strangers' house looking at their personal items but looking back now, I wouldn't change it for the world. That encounter is ultimately the motivation behind The Gluten Free Awards and the associated Gluten Free Buyers Guide. We left her house with complete understanding of cross contamination, best practices and what products they personally liked and disliked. That visit was life changing and left us feeling confident as we made our way to the local health food store.

That first trip shopping took forever. Each label was read and cross checked with our list of known gluten containing suspects. It was also shocking to see the bill when it was time to pay. We had replaced our entire pantry and fridge with all products that had the "Gluten Free" label. We both worked full-time and had decent paying jobs and it still set us back financially.

We looked for support groups locally and came across a "100% Gluten-Free Picnic" in Raleigh, which was two hours away from where we lived. This was our first time meeting other people with celiac disease and we were fortunate to have met some informative people that were willing to help with the hundreds of questions we had. We were introduced to a family whose son had been recently diagnosed with celiac disease as well. His condition was much worse than Jacobs and he was almost hospitalized before finally being diagnosed. They confided in us as we shared similar stories. There were two differences that would change my life forever. The first was the fact that they didn't have the same experience with a registered dietitian. Instead they were handed a two-page Xerox copy of "safe foods". Second, they didn't have the financial security to experiment with gluten free counterparts. Their first two months exposed to the gluten free life style left them extremely depressed and broke.

On our way home from that picnic, Jayme and I felt compelled to help make a difference in some way. We were determined to help that family and others being diagnosed with this disease. Up until that day, we hadn't found a resource that gave unbiased opinions on gluten free products and services. Fast forward a few years and I too was diagnosed with celiac disease. That year, The Gluten Free Awards were born.

Originally our vision was to create a one-page website with a handful of categories organized by peoples' favorites. Since 2010 we have produced The Annual Gluten Free Awards (GFA) growing into sixty gluten free categories. After several requests, in 2014, we took the GFA results and published our first Gluten Free Buyers Guide. The annual guide is sold primarily in the United States however we continue to see increased global sales. Each year we have over 3,000 people vote for their favorite gluten free products and we now communicate to nearly 20,000 people weekly through our email list and social media channels.

We want to thank those special people and organizations that brought us to where we are today:

Pat Fogarty MS, RD, LDN for allowing us to enter your home.

Jeff Gordon's Children's Hospital

Raleigh Celiac Support Groups

Rebecca Panuski, MD

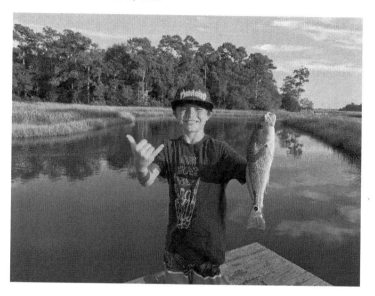

I hope you have learned something new from the story behind The Gluten Free Awards. Today, Jacob and I continue to live a healthy gluten free lifestyle.

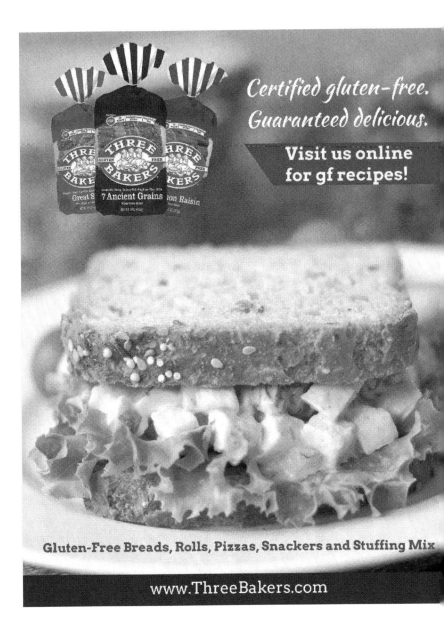

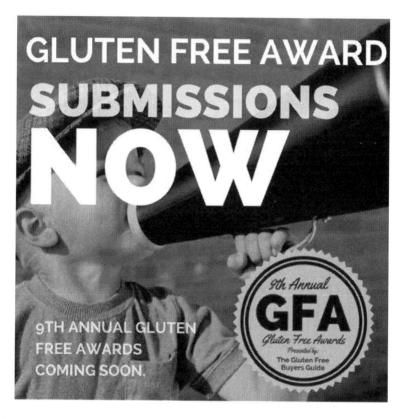

Learn more on page 174

Best Gluten Free Bagels

8th Annual Gluten-Free Awards:
1st Place: Canyon Bakehouse Gluten Free Blueberry Bagels

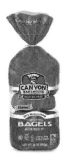

2nd Place: Against the Grain Sesame Bagels

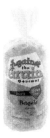

3rd Place: Katz Gluten Free, English Muffins

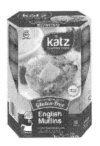

Other Nominees:

Franz Gluten Free Plain Bagels

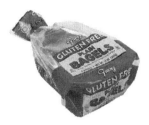

Barely Bread the onion-garlic-sea salt 100% Grain-Free Bagel

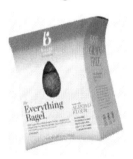

Promise Gluten-Free Plain Bagels

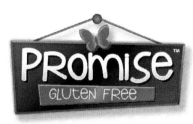

Best Gluten Free Beer Brands

8th Annual Gluten-Free Awards:

1st Place: Ghostfish Brewing Company

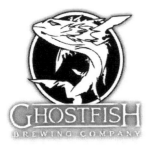

2nd Place: Redbridge

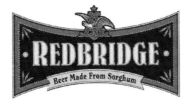

3rd Place: Glutenberg

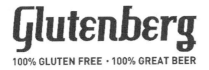

Other Nominees:

Green's

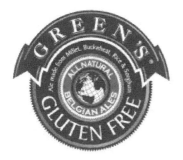

Bards

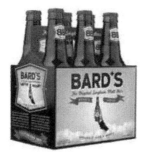

Ground Breaker Brewing

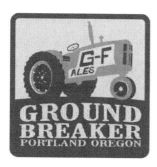

Best Gluten Free Blogs

8th Annual Gluten-Free Awards:

1st Place: GF Jules

http://gfjules.com/

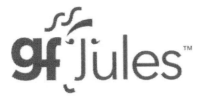

2nd Place: Gluten-Free on a Shoestring

http://glutenfreeonashoestring.com/

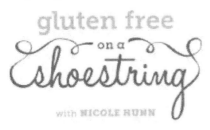

3rd Place: Simply Gluten Free

http://simplygluten-free.com/

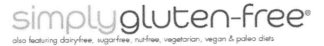

Other nominees:

Gluten Dude

What The Fork Food Blog

Celiac & The Beast

Gluten Free Girl

Living Freely Gluten Free

Gluten Free Globetrotter

Gluten Free Follow Me

Gluten Free Goddess

Elenas Pantry

I'm a Celiac

Tasty Mediation

Vegetarian Mamma

Hannah Ross Crane

King Gluten Free

Gluten Free Palate

Gluten Free Ireland

Strength and Sunshine

Best Gluten Free Books

8th Annual Gluten-Free Awards:

1st Place: The First Year: Celiac Disease and Living Gluten-Free: An Essential Guide for the Newly Diagnosed: Jules Shepard

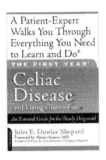

2nd Place: Gluten Is My Bitch: Rants, Recipes, and Ridiculousness for the Gluten-Free by April Peveteaux

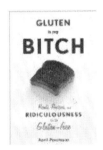

3rd Place: Jennifer's Way: My Journey with Celiac Disease--What Doctors Don't Tell You and How You Can Learn to Live Again by Jennifer Esposito

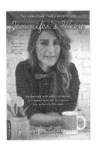

Other Nominees:

Celiac and the Beast: A Love Story Between a Gluten-Free Girl, Her Genes, and a Broken Digestive Tract by Erica Dermer

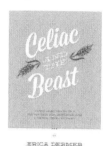

Gluten Freedom: The Nation's Leading Expert Offers the Essential Guide to a Healthy, Gluten-Free Lifestyle by Alessio Fasano (Author), Susie Flaherty (Contributor)

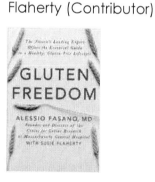

The Celiac Cookbook and Survival Guide by Pam Jordan

Dough Nation by Nadine Grzeskowiak

Gluten Free Fork: A collection of 40 simple to make, budget-friendly recipes to nourish your family by Cindy Gordon

Best Gluten Free Bread Brands

8th Annual Gluten-Free Awards:
1st Place: Canyon Bakehouse 7-Grain Bread

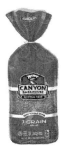

2nd Place: Three Bakers 7 Ancient Grains Whole Grain Bread

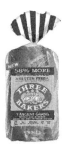

3rd Place: Schär Artisan Baker White Bread

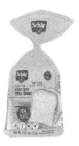

Other nominees:

Schär: Artisan Baker Multigrain Bread

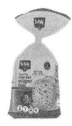

Three Bakers Great Seed Whole Grain and 7 Seed Bread

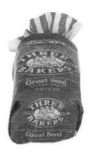

Franz Gluten Free 7 Grain

Three Bakers White Bread Whole Grain

ALDI liveGfree White Gluten Free Bread

ADLI liveGfree Whole Grain Gluten Free Bread

Bread SRSLY Classic Sourdough

BFree - Brown Seeded Sandwich Loaf

Best Gluten Free Bread Crumbs

8th Annual Gluten-Free Awards:

1st Placer: Glutino Bread Crumbs

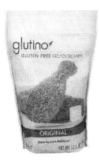

2nd Place: Schar Gluten Free Bread Crumbs

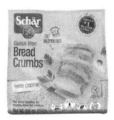

3rd Place: Aleia's Gluten Free Foods Bread Crumbs

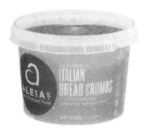

Other nominees:

Katz Gluten Free Bread Crumbs

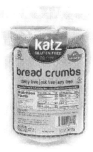

Gillian's Foods Gluten Free Italian Bread Crumbs

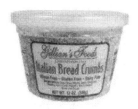

Watusee Foods Chickpea Crumbs

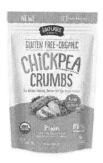

Article: Why Do I Need a Celiac Diagnosis?

By: Erica Dermer

I always get the question "why do I need a celiac diagnosis?" This is usually because people think because non-celiac gluten sensitivity (now called non-celiac wheat sensitivity) and a celiac both eat the same diet, that they are the same condition. Why bother with all the tests if you eat the same anyways? Because celiac is some serious shit. It's the difference between my lactose intolerance and my celiac disease. Because I know that every bite of something made with butter instead of oil can be helped by digestive enzymes and won't really affect me that horribly. I won't get cancer from it. I won't become infertile from it. I won't have GERD and gastroparesis so bad I'll throw up on a stranger because of it. I won't become a raging bitch because of it and turn into the Incredible Hulk. Because it's an intolerance. It's not an autoimmune disease.

At this point, I'll get people writing in saying "how dare you!" Yes, I acknowledge that non-celiac gluten intolerance is a very real thing and it's awful. Yes, we all eat the same, but how we control and take care of the issues because of it are different. I am not calling your issues fake or belittling you. It's just a different thing.

I am a proponent of getting properly tested. I care about getting properly tested because I wasn't at first, and they thought it was a million other things besides celiac. If I had gone with my first diagnosis I'd still be 40 pounds less and still eating gluten.

It's incredibly important to get a formal diagnosis via an endoscopy after a blood screening test.This is currently a gold standard for diagnosis.

"But a blood test can have a false positive/false negative/equivocal results!" Yes it can! And way too many people don't realize that they have to be eating a ton of gluten while having the blood test or else it won't show anything. My blood tests didn't really show anything, I had to combine with multiple endoscopies and a blood test along with symptomology to really see if I was celiac. And yes, I had to go back on eating gluten for these endoscopies and blood tests. Back on the thing that gave me rashes and made my mouth an open sore. That made me cry and act like a crazy teen going through hormonal changes. But I did it.

So what if you're not eating gluten anymore and refuse to be tested? TOUGH COOKIES. Either go on a gluten-containing diet for 6-12 weeks and have an endoscopy or don't. But if you don't, there is no gold standard diagnosis without it. You doctor can put together pieces with other information, positive serology, positive genetic test (you don't need to be eating gluten for that), symptoms while on gluten and probably give you a diagnosis, but this is only if you have a really good GI that has ruled out other things. Celiac is an imitator, you can have a myriad of other issues like Crohn's, colitis, IBS, a million other things besides celiac. So it's good to know if this is really it.

But most importantly, in my opinion, is what you do after the diagnosis. It's really just a starting point once you get diagnosed. You need to have the following follow-up 1) bone density screening 2) nutritional deficiency screening 3) follow-up endoscopy to see if you are healing properly 4) follow-up for additional autoimmune disease. If you don't have celiac, this isn't something you need to worry about. But if you do get diagnosed with celiac, it's important to start healing and make sure you're healing properly with this follow-up protocol. Celiac ravages your body. Make sure you schedule proper follow-ups, and if need be – get a new doctor who cares about following up with your celiac disease. You have this disease forever, don't forget about it the second you go on a gluten-free diet.

Gluten Free Humor

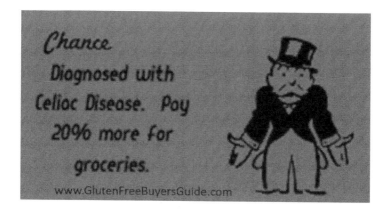

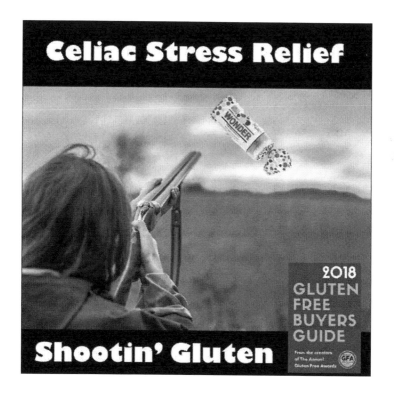

Best Gluten Free Bread Mixes

8th Annual Gluten-Free Awards:

1st Place: gfJules Bread Mix

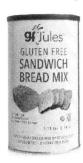

2nd Place: Bob's Red Mill - Homemade Wonderful Bread Mix

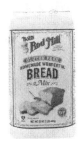

3rd Place: Pamela's Products Gluten-free Bread Mix

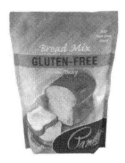

Other nominees:

Chebe Bread Mix

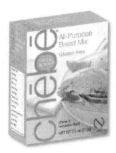

Simple Mills Artisan Bread Mix

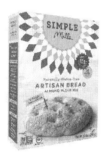

Luce's Gluten Free Artisan Bread Mix

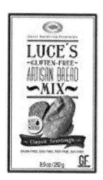

Best Gluten Free Breakfast On-The-Go

8th Annual Gluten-Free Awards:

1st Place: Pamela's Products Gluten Free Whenever Bars, Oat Chocolate Chip Coconut

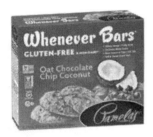

2nd Place: Glutino Gluten Free Strawberry Toaster Pastries

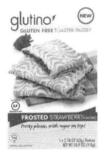

3rd Place: Bob's Red Mill Gluten Free Apple Cinnamon Oatmeal Cup

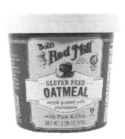

Other nominees:

Luna Bar Gluten Free, Lemon Zest

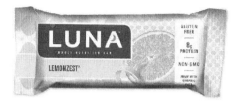

ALDI liveGfree Gluten Free Cocoa Loco Baked Chewy Bars

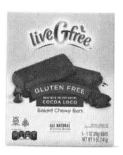

Enjoy Life Cranberry Orange ProBurst Bites

ALDI liveGfree Gluten Free Baked Very Berry Chewy Bars

ALDI liveGfree Gluten Free Caramel Apple Baked Chewy Bars

KNOW Foods Gluten Free Protein Bars, Low Carb, Paleo + Keto Friendly

ProYo High Protein Frozen Yogurt

Best Gluten Free Brownie Mix

8th Annual Gluten-Free Awards:

1st Place: gfJules Brownie Mix

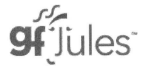

2nd Place: King Arthur Flour Gluten Free Brownie Mix

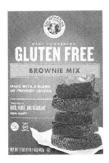

3rd Place: Pamela's Products Gluten Free Chocolate Brownie Mix

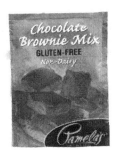

Other Nominees:

Duncan Hines Gluten-Free Brownies

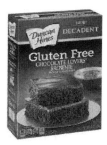

Enjoy Life Brownie Mix

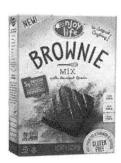

Gluten-Free Prairie Deep Dark Chocolate Brownie Mix

Glutino Brownie Mix

Better Batter Brownie Mix

Best Gluten Free Buns

8th Annual Gluten-Free Awards:
1st Place: Canyon Bakehouse Gluten Free Hamburger Buns

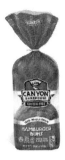

2nd Place: Udi's Gluten Free Classic Hamburger Buns

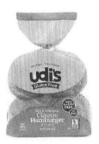

3rd Place: Schar Gluten Free Hamburger Buns

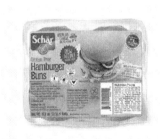

Other Nominees:

Three Bakers Whole Grain Hamburger Buns

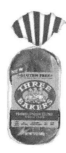

Franz Gluten Free Hamburger Buns

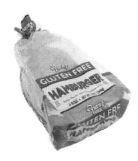

Three Bakers Whole Grain Hot Dog Buns

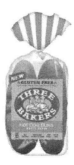

Little Norther Bakehouse Millet & Chia Buns

Best Gluten Free Cake Mix

8th Annual Gluten-Free Awards:

1st Place: Pillsbury - Gluten-Free Funfetti Mix

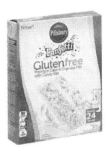

2nd Place: Pamela's Products Gluten Free Cake Mix Classic Vanilla

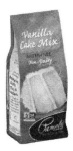

3rd Place: Bob's Red Mill Gluten Free Chocolate Cake Mix

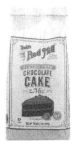

Other Nominees:

Aldi liveGfree Gluten Free Yellow Baking Mix

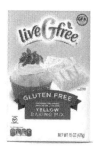

Better Batter Cake Mix Gluten Free Yellow

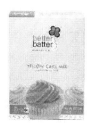

123 Gluten Free Delightfully Gratifying Poundcake Mix Hint of Lemon

123 Gluten Free Sweet Goodness Pan Bars Mix

Article: The Birthday Party Hangover

by Celiac Mama, Jereann Zann, mother to a fun-loving 4 year old who has celiac disease and a dairy allergy.

Many of us associate a birthday hangover as something that adults experience after drinking too much at a party the night before. However, when you have a child that has celiac disease or a gluten/dairy allergy it takes on another meaning. They see their friends eating birthday cake, treats, candy in party favor bags and often pizza and they can't participate. Yes, we do our best to bring gluten free and allergy friendly treats so that our children have something yummy to eat, but it's not the same as being part of the group. So, often times, the next day we see sadness, low self esteem due to feeling left out or different – what we have come to call the "birthday party hangover".

Let me first say, it's totally normal for your child to experience these feelings. Second, even with these feelings our daughter always wants to go to birthday parties to see her friends and celebrate. So, since our daughter loves parties and we want her to be able to participate as much as possible, we've developed some strategies that I hope will help you too.

Before the Party:

Call the parent hosting the party to find out as much about the food being served as possible so that you can bring similar safe treats for your little one.

Birthday Party Hangover Cure:

In four words – fun in the kitchen! It is so important for your child to have a positive relationship with food – it reduces stigma, anxiety, and depression. So, the next day to combat the hangover, get your child in the kitchen and make something together.

Was there something that he/she saw at the birthday party that they want to try? Perfect, make that. Or if not, is there something that they've been talking about a lot (i.e. donuts, chocolate, cookies) that you know they would enjoy? In our experience, making it dessert related is the way to go, but pizza is a big hit too. Let your child get messy, let him/her really get involved in the preparation and of course the eating once it's ready. Make it fun, play music, get matching aprons, etc. so that it becomes an exciting tradition in your house.

Having fun in the kitchen not only distracts them from feeling blue, but it also shows them that they don't have to live WITHOUT. It teaches them that they can have those things too, just prepared differently so that it's safe for them to eat. This will also assist with opening up communication lines so that they tell you if someone else's snack or lunch at school looked good, and hopefully reduce snack sharing.

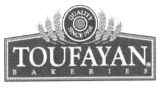

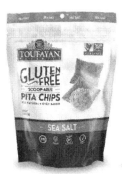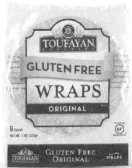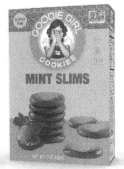

DID YOU KNOW?

30-50% OF WORLD POPULATION HAS GENETIC PREDISPOSITION TO CELIAC DISEASE

Quoted from:
17th International Celiac Disease
Symposium in New Delhi, India

Best Gluten Free Children's Book

8th Annual Gluten-Free Awards:

1st Place: Eat Like a Dinosaur: Recipe & Guidebook for Gluten-free Kids by Paleo Parents and Elana Amsterdam

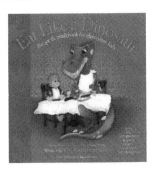

2nd Place: The GF Kid: A Celiac Disease Survival Guide by Melissa London and Eric Glickman

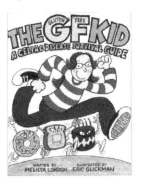

3rd Place: Eating Gluten-Free with Emily: A Story for Children with Celiac Disease by Bonnie J. Kruszka and Richard S. Cihlar

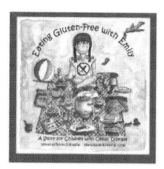

Other nominees:

Santa's Gluten Free Cookie Plate: Timeless Traditional Recipes by Tiffany Hinton

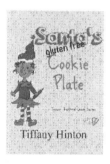

Adam's Gluten Free Surprise: Helping Others Understand Gluten Free by Debbie Simpson

Gordy and the Magic Diet by by Kim Diersen (Author), April Runge (Author), Carrie Hartman (Illustrator)

The Gluten Glitch by Stasie John and Kevin Cannon

Best Gluten Free Chips

8th Annual Gluten-Free Awards:

1st Place: POPCORNERS Carnival Kettle, Popped Corn Chips, Gluten Free, Non-GMO

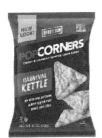

2nd Place: Way Better Snacks Sprouted Gluten Free Tortilla Chips Unbeatable Blues

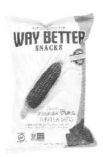

3rd Place: ALDI liveGfree Black Sesame Brown Rice Crisps

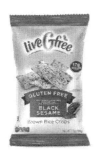

Other Nominees:

Beanfields Bean and Rice Chips – Nacho

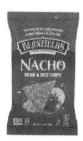

ALDI liveGfree Sweet Chili Brown Rice Crisps

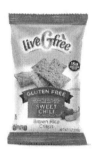

Toufayan Gluten Free Pita Chips - Sea Salt

Saffron Road Chickbean Crisps, Sea Salt

Simply 7 BBQ Quinoa Chips

RW Garcia Yellow & Blue Corn MixtBag Tortilla Chips

Toufayan Gluten Free Pita Chips - Chili Lime

RW Garcia Veggie & White Corn MixtBag Tortilla Chips

Best Gluten Free Cold Cereal

8th Annual Gluten-Free Awards:

1st Place: Corn Chex

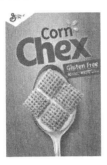

2nd Place: Envirokidz Organic Leapin' Lemurs Peanut Butter and Chocolate Cereal

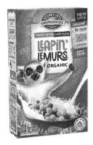

3rd Place: Bob's Red Mill Gluten Free Tropical Muesli

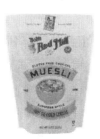

Other nominees:

Gluten-Free Prairie Montana Mornings Granola

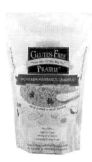

Freedom Foods Gluten Free Cereal Tropicos

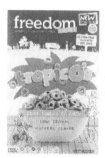

Love Grown Fruity Sea Stars

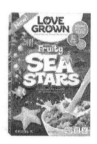

Best Gluten Free Accommodating Colleges

8th Annual Gluten-Free Awards:

1st Place: UNIVERSITY OF COLORADO: BOULDER

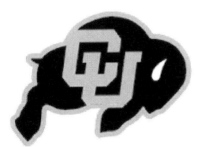

2nd Place: OREGON STATE UNIVERSITY

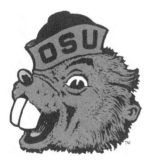

3rd Place: SAN DIEGO STATE

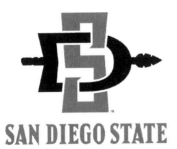

Other nominees:

KENT STATE UNIVERSITY

UNIVERSITY OF ARIZONA

UNIVERSITY OF NOTRE DAME

UNIVERSITY OF TENNESSEE

UNIVERSITY OF CONNECTICUT

IOWA STATE UNIVERSITY

NC STATE UNIVERSITY

ITHACA COLLEGE

YALE UNIVERSITY

UNIVERSITY OF NEW HAMPSHIRE

GEORGETOWN UNIVERSITY

COLUMBIA UNIVERSITY

TOWSON UNIVERSITY

CARLETON COLLEGE

CLARK UNIVERSITY

Best Gluten Free Comfort Food

8th Annual Gluten-Free Awards:

1st Place: Glutino Yogurt Covered Pretzels

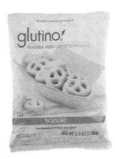

2nd Place: Amy's Mac n Cheese

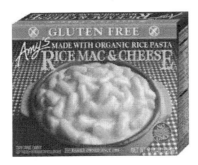

3rd Place: Mary's Gone Crackers Lightly Salted Thins

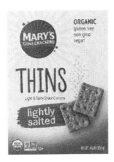

Other nominees:

Daiya Mac and Cheese

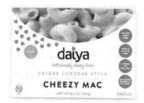

Nibmor Dark Chocolate with Cherries Bar

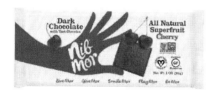

Dr. Praeger's Rice Crusted Fish Sticks

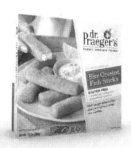

Boulder Organic Foods Chicken Noodle Soup

Le Veneziane Lasagne

Banza Mac and Cheese

Best Gluten Free Cookbooks

8th Annual Gluten-Free Awards:

1st Place: Free for All Cooking: 150 Easy Gluten-Free, Allergy-Friendly Recipes the Whole Family Can Enjoy by Jules E. Dowler Shepard

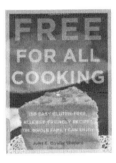

2nd Place : Nearly Normal Cooking For Gluten-Free Eating: A Fresh Approach to Cooking and Living Without Wheat or Gluten by Jules E. D. Shepard

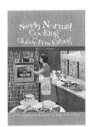

3rd Place: The How Can It Be Gluten Free Cookbook Paperback by America's Test Kitchen (Editor)

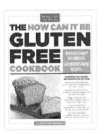

Other nominees:

Danielle Walker's Against All Grain Celebrations: A Year of Gluten-Free, Dairy-Free, and Paleo Recipes for Every Occasion by Danielle Walker

Gluten-Free Makeovers: Over 175 Recipes--from Family Favorites to Gourmet Goodies--Made Deliciously Wheat-Free by Beth Hillson

The Easy Gluten-Free Cookbook: Fast and Fuss-Free Recipes for Busy People on a Gluten-Free Diet by Lindsay Garza

The Warm Kitchen by Amy Fothergill by Amy Fothergill

Clean Eating with a Dirty Mind: Over 150 Paleo-Inspired Recipes for Every Craving by Vanessa Barajas and Juli Bauer

Gluten Free Fork: A collection of 40 simple to make, budget-friendly recipes to nourish your family by Cindy Gordon

Sweet & Simple Gluten-Free Baking: Irresistible Classics in 10 Ingredients or Less! by Chrystal Carver

Bread & Butter: Gluten-Free Vegan Recipes to Fill Your Bread Basket by Erin McKenna

Family Approved Gluten Free Recipes by Pam Jordan

Beautiful Smoothie Bowls: 80 Delicious and Colorful Superfood Recipes to Nourish and Satisfy by Carissa Bonham

Best Gluten Free Cookie Mixes

8th Annual Gluten-Free Awards:

1st Place: gfJules Original Cookie Mix

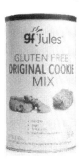

2nd Place: Betty Crocker Gluten-Free Chocolate Chip Mix

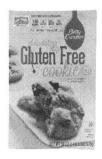

3rd Place   Pamela's Chocolate Chip Cookie Mix

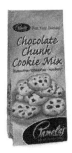

Other nominees:

Immaculate Baking Gluten Free Cookie Mix Sugar

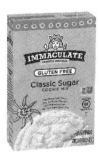

Hodgson Mill Gluten Free Cookie Mix

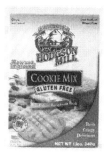

Simple Mills Chocolate Chip Cookie

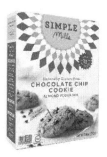

123 Gluten Free Lindsay's Lipsmackin' Sugar Cookie Mix

Best Gluten Free Cookies

8th Annual Gluten-Free Awards:

1st Place: Tate's Chocolate Chip

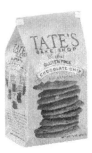

2nd Place: Goodie Girl Cookies – Mint Slims

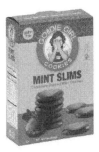

3rd Place: Enjoy Life Soft Baked Cookies, Gluten-Free, Dairy- Free, Nut-Free and Soy-Free, Double Chocolate Brownie

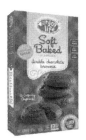

Other nominees:

Enjoy Life Foods Soft Bake Snickerdoodle

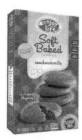

Schär: Honeygrams

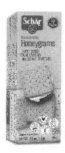

Schär: Chocolate Dipped Cookies

ALDI liveGfree Gluten Free Snickerdoodle Soft Baked Cookies

ALDI liveGfree Gluten Free Double Chocolate Brownie Soft Baked Cookies

Gluten-Free Prairie Hunger Buster Cookie

Goodie Girl Cookies – Chocolate Chunk

Best Gluten Free Cornbread Mix

8th Annual Gluten-Free Awards:

1st Place: gfJules Cornbread Mix

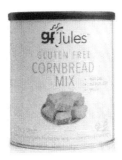

2nd Place: Krusteaz Gluten Free Honey Cornbread Mix

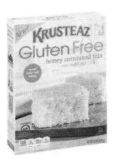

3rd Place: Bob's Red Mill Gluten Free Cornbread Mix

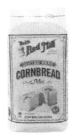

Other nominees:

Pamela's Gluten Free Cornbread Mix

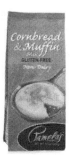

Glutino Cornbread Mix

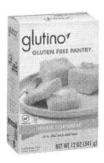

Best Gluten Free Cosmetic Brands

8th Annual Gluten-Free Awards:

1st Place: tarte

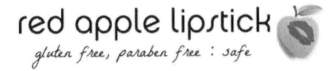

2nd Place: Red Apple Lipstick

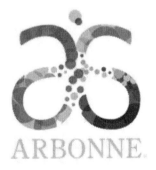

3rd Place: Arbonne

Other nominees:

Afterglow

Au Naturale

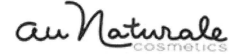

Kiss Freely

ILIA Beauty

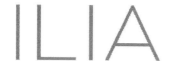

Venus Skin

Article: A Roundup of Gluten Free Beauty Products

Hannah Ross Crane, Huffington Post Contributor & Assistant Director, NYU Law Institute for Executive Education

Finding gluten free cosmetics can be one of the trickiest challenges to overcome when you have celiac disease. About two years ago I wrote an article titled Is Gluten Hiding in Your Beauty Routine? At the time I was still learning about what products were safe and which were not, and so I figured that I would do an updated, comprehensive, gluten free cosmetic roundup with truly trustworthy brands that I love and use every day.

Some people might be thinking to themselves, "but if I don't eat my shampoo, what's the problem?" Well, if you have ever been able to successfully shower without having some water run down your face my hat is off to you! It's a really difficult feat to accomplish! I for one have not been able to do this, and so gluten free shampoo puts my mind at ease.

As far as other body products go it is critical to maintain a fully gluten free lifestyle in order to prevent any possible cross contamination. Soaps and lotions often end up on your hands- so if you touch your mouth or eat some finger foods, going gluten free with those products is a good idea.

Additionally, some people have Dermatitis herpetiformis- also known as DH or Duhring's Disease. Defined by celiac.org as "...a skin manifestation of non-celiac wheat sensitivity," DH causes "...extremely itchy bumps or blisters [that] appear on both sides of the body, most often on the forearms near the elbows, as well as on knees and buttocks, and along the hairline." Many people with DH use gluten free products to reduce and address their symptoms.

A gentle reminder for those out there who think celiac disease just means getting a stomach ache when an individual is exposed to gluten- this is not the case. In addition to possible gastrointestinal discomfort, gluten exposure can result in increased risk for cancer, other autoimmune diseases, neurological problems, and infertility.

With all of that out of the way, here is my list of products that I swear by. I hope you enjoy them and that this helps you on your journey back to health!

Acure Organics: Acure Organics has amazing shampoos, conditioners, body washes, face oils, serums, and lotions among a wide array of other products. I use their shampoo and conditioner, as well as their argan oil every day!

Andalou Naturals: Andalou Naturals carries a number of lotions, hair products, body butters, and more. They even have some amazing sheet masks which are a favorite indulgence of mine!

EO Products: EO has almost anything you could dream of. According to their website, EO stands for "essential oils" which is where the company's journey began. Personally, I rely on them for their essential oils and bath products. EO bubble baths, bath salts, and soaks are particularly heavenly!

Everyone Products: Everyone Products are an offshoot of EO Products and are FANTASTIC! According to the website, Everyone Products is "...a line of products designed for young people and large families who [have] little or no choice for quality, botanical body products." They are designed to be body, earth, and budget friendly! I have a bottle of their hand soap next to every sink in my apartment and I regularly use their Epsom Salt Bath soaks. I love that they also have a certified gluten free line of baby products!

Ilia Beauty: I rarely use makeup, but every now and then I reach for a concealer. When I was first diagnosed with celiac disease finding a brand of concealer that fit my needs was incredibly challenging. In addition to celiac disease I have a number of chemical allergies and allergies to common makeup ingredients like avocado and almond oil (the latter two have since disappeared, yay!) but Ilia Beauty was, and still is, an absolute lifesaver for me. Their products are all certified gluten free and cruelty free!

Red Apple Lipstick: Despite their renowned lipsticks, I really only use the Red Apple Lipstick mascara (for special occasions!). However their lipstick selection is out of sight and a must for anyone with celiac disease.

Kiss Freely: I rely on Kiss Freely for their lip balm selection. These products are all free of the 8 major allergens. Additionally, they avoid using sesame, shea butter, peas, coconut, avocado, and sunflower seed. Needless to say they are another lifesaver for me. They are also a family company founded by the mother of a young woman with severe food allergies. A wonderful company with amazing products and a mission that hits home is exactly the kind of business I want to be supporting.

MyChelle Dermaceuticals: Sunscreen is a critical part of anyone's beauty regimen, but when you have celiac disease finding a truly safe brand is actually very difficult. MyChelle is my brand of choice when it comes to sunscreen. Their Sun Shield SPF 28 sunscreen in Coconut is my favorite! It smells just like a tropical vacation! Also, their sunscreens don't leave you as white and streaky as other natural brands which is definitely a plus!

These are just a few of my favorite brands with products that I use, have vetted, and can wholeheartedly swear by. I hope this list is helpful to you. If you have any questions, stories, or favorite products you would like to share I welcome you to comment below or share them with me at hannah.crane@nyu.edu.

*Disclaimer: All opinions presented are my own. I was not paid or compensated to endorse any party mentioned in this article. *

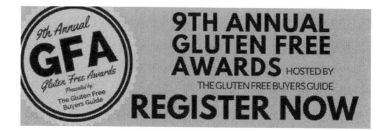

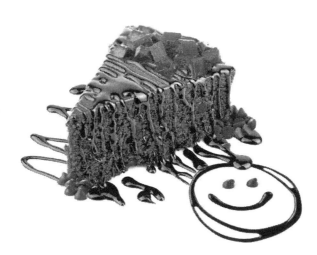

PURE DELIGHT

NO SOY · NO DAIRY · ALL CHOCOLATE

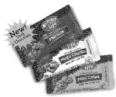

Make the deliciously sweet and safe choice with Enjoy Life **Semi-Sweet Mini Chips, Mega Chunks** and **NEW Dark Morsels**! They're dairy and nut free as well as free from the 8 most common allergens, and because we don't use soy fillers, there's room for more pure chocolate! All our chocolate is created in a dedicated nut free facility, so you can eat freely while enjoying every bit of chocolate decadence.

EAT FREELY, ENJOY FULLY

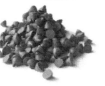

Learn more about our complete line of delicious Free-From products at

enjoylifefoods.com   #eatfreely

DID YOU KNOW?

CELIAC DISEASE: INCREASED TO 3% IN US (NOT 1% AS CONSISTENTLY REPORTED)

Quoted from:
17th International Celiac Disease
Symposium in New Delhi, India

Best Gluten Free Crackers

8th Annual Gluten-Free Awards:

1st Place: Schär Table Crackers

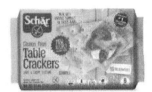

2nd Place: Mary's Gone Crackers - Super Seed Classic Crackers

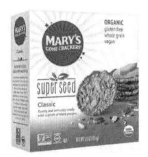

3rd Place: ALDI liveGfree Gluten Free Sea Salt Multi Seed Cracker

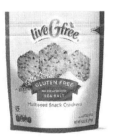

Other nominees:

Mary's Gone Crackers - Herb Crackers

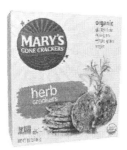

Simple Mills Fine Ground Sea Salt Almond Flour Crackers

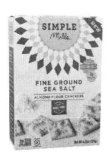

Absolutely Gluten Free Crackers

Simple Mills Farmhouse Cheddar Almond Flour Crackers

Saffron Road Rosemary Lentil Crackers

RW Garcia 3 Seed Sweet Potato Crackers

Le Veneziane Grissini

RW Garcia 3 Seed Sweet Beet Crackers

RW Garcia 3 Seed Kale Crackers

Best Gluten Free Donuts

8th Annual Gluten-Free Awards:

1st Place: Katz Gluten Free, Glazed Donuts

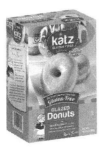

2nd Place: Kinnikinnick Wheat Free Glazed Donut, Maple

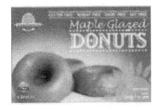

3rd Place: Katz Gluten Free, Powdered Donuts

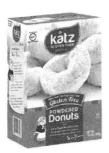

Other Nominees:

Katz Gluten Free, Glazed Chocolate Donut Holes

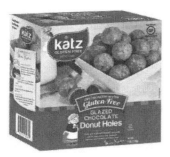

Bare Naked Bakery Donuts

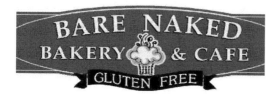

KNOW Better Donuts

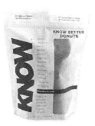

Best Gluten Free Expo and Events

8th Annual Gluten-Free Awards:

1st Place: Gluten & Allergen Free Expos

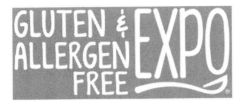

2nd Place: Living Without's Gluten Free Food Allergy Fest

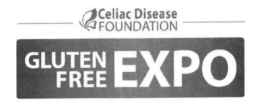

3rd Place: T CDF National Education & Gluten-Free Expo

Other nominees:

Gluten & Allergen Free Wellness Events

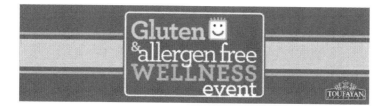

Natural Products Expo West

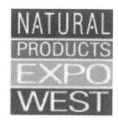

Natural Products Expo East

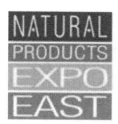

Best Gluten Free Flours

8th Annual Gluten-Free Awards:

1st Place: gfJules Gluten Free All Purpose Flour

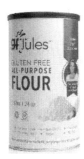

2nd Place: Bob's Red Mill 1-to-1

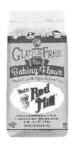

3rd Place: Better Batter Gluten-Free Flour

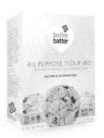

Other nominees:

Glutino Gluten-Free Pantry All Purpose Baking Flour

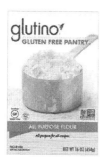

Enjoy Life All-Purpose Flour

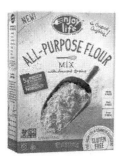

Gluten-Free Prairie Simply Wholesome All Purpose Flour Blend

Gluten-Free Prairie Toasted Oat Flour

Premium Organic Tiger Nuts Flour

Pereg Natural Foods Multi-Purpose Alternative Gluten Free Banana Flour, All-Natural, Non-GMO, Kosher, Vegan

Recipe: Pumpkin Donuts with Maple Glaze- Gluten Free, Dairy Free

By Jennifer Bigler at livingfreelyglutenfree.com

Donuts are hands down the one thing I miss the most since going gluten free. If you follow me, then you hear me talk about donuts a lot. That's why these gluten free and dairy free pumpkin donuts with maple glaze are a huge hit in my house.

We all have that one food we miss. It's the one thing that makes us weak in the knees and that tests our will power. For me, that one thing is donuts. I miss them so freaking bad. My cake donuts like Funfetti with Strawberry Glaze and Chocolate are definitely a great way to curb that craving. However, a true yeast risen donut is still on my mind (like all the freaking time) so, I plan to work on that one soon. I know it is going to be quite the task, so I am waiting for some free time, that way I can really tackle it.

These pumpkin donuts are VERY easy and fast to make! You will need a Donut Baking Pan. For years I have been using a regular Wilton pan, and they work fine, but I just purchased silicon donut pans-OMG, game changer. These are so much easier to use and clean up WAY faster than a traditional pan. These are the exact Donut Baking Panones I have and I highly recommend them.

This batter is super simple to make, and the donuts bake fast. I use a cookie sheet under the silicon donut pan to make life easier, please do it! Line a cooling rack with parchment paper. After the donuts are done, let them sit for 5 minutes and then turn the silicon pan upside down on top of your parchment paper and pop them out. I use a little coconut oil to grease the pan. You can easily nudge them out if they need a little help just by pushing on the mold. Let them cool completely before frosting.

Cake donuts always taste best when eaten the day of baking. With all of my donut recipes, I recommend not frosting until you are ready to serve. Once you frost them, let them sit for 30 minutes before serving. This gives the glaze an opportunity to firm up slightly and be less messy. With all of my donut recipes, you can always bake the day before and then frost before serving the next day. You can freeze unfrosted donuts as well. If you don't plan on eating an entire batch, then just cut the frosting recipe in half, and freeze the remaining donuts.

These will majorly impress at a brunch, holiday breakfast, or afternoon tea. I however, just eat them because I want to. My kids even went crazy for them and they are partial to chocolate desserts. These donuts are a winner and will be your favorite fall treat!

Yields: 18 Donuts

Ingredients:

2 Eggs

¾ Cup Sugar

1 tsp. Vanilla

1 Cup Brown Sugar

1 Cup Pureed Pumpkin

1 Cup Dairy Free Milk (I used coconut)

3 tsp. Baking Powder

2 Cups GF All Purpose Flour

1 tsp. Xanthan Gum

1 tsp. Pumpkin Pie Spice

Dash of Salt

1 tsp. Cinnamon

¼ tsp. Nutmeg

Glaze:

2 Cups Powdered Sugar

1 ½ tsp. Vanilla

½ tsp. Cinnamon

½ tsp. Maple Extract Maple Extract

2 ½ TBSP. Coconut Milk (any dairy free milk will do)

Directions

1.   Preheat your oven to 350°F.

2.   In a stand mixer, cream the eggs with the sugar and vanilla.

3.   Once creamed, add the pumpkin and dairy free milk while the stand mixer is on low.

4.   Add the baking powder, xanthan gum, all the spices and salt.

5.   Beat for one minute and then add the GF all-purpose flour.

6.   On medium speed, beat for an additional 5 minutes scraping down the sides halfway through. Grease your donut pan (I use coconut oil) and then spoon the batter in.

7.   Bake for about 20 minutes or until a toothpick comes out clean.

8.   Once done, allow the donut pan to sit for 5 minutes. Transfer the donuts onto a cooling rack lined with parchment paper and allow to completely cool before frosting.

Glaze:

1.   In a bowl whisk together all of the ingredients until the glaze is smooth. Drop the donuts directly into the glaze and pick up with one finger. Lay the donuts glaze side up on parchment paper and allow to sit for 30 minutes before serving.

For best flavor frost before serving.

Best Gluten Free Frozen Meals

8th Annual Gluten-Free Awards:

1st Place: Amy's Rice Macaroni & Cheese, Gluten-Free

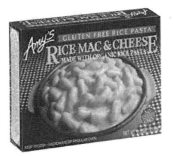

2nd Place: Evol Fire Grilled Steak Bowl

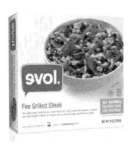

3rd Place: Gluten Free Delights - Uncured Pepperoni Pizza

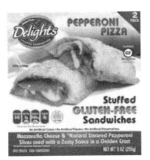

Other nominees:

Udi's Broccoli and Kale Lasagna

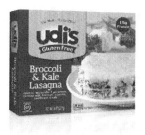

Dr. Praeger's California Veggie Burgers

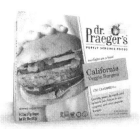

Saffron Road Korean-Style Sweet Chili Chicken Bowl

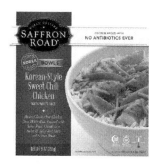

FEEL GOOD FOODS Entre Mongolian Beef with Asparagus

Best Gluten Free Frozen Pancake & Waffle Brands

8th Annual Gluten-Free Awards:

1st Place: Van's Gluten Free Waffles

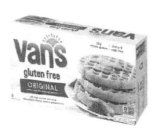

2nd Place: Trader Joe's Gluten-Free Waffles

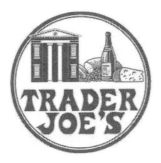

3rd Place: Nature's Path Homestyle Frozen Waffle

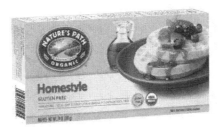

Other Nominees:

Kashi Gluten Free Waffles

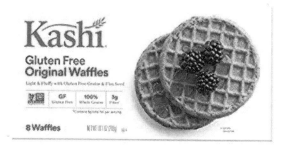

Know Foods Gluten Free Waffles

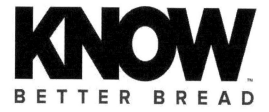

Best Gluten Free Frozen Pizza Brands

8th Annual Gluten-Free Awards:

1st Place: Freschetta Pepperoni Pizza

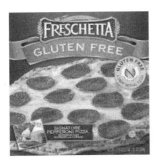

2nd Place: Three Bakers Classic Cheese Thin Crust Pizza

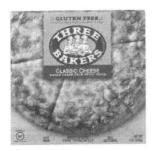

3rd Place: Daiya Cheeze Lover's Pizza

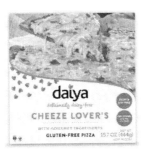

Other nominees:

Three Bakers Mild Pepperoni Thin Crust Pizza

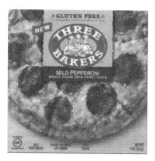

Sonoma Flatbread Uncured Pepperoni

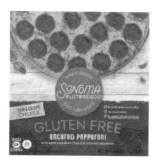

Three Bakers Sweet Italian Sausage Thin Crust Pizza

Califlour Foods (Crust)

Smart Flour Foods; Uncured Pepperoni Pizza

Spinato's Tomato Basil Garlic

Spinato's Mozzeralla Cheese

Spinato's Pepperoni

Best Gluten Free Granola

8th Annual Gluten-Free Awards:

1st Place: KIND Healthy Grains Granola Clusters, Peanut Butter Whole Grain, Gluten Free

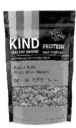

2nd Place: Bakery On Main's Bakery On Main Gluten-Free, Non GMO Granola, Cranberry Almond Maple

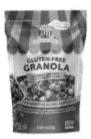

3rd Place: Purely Elizabeth Ancient Grain Granola, Original

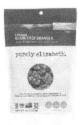

Other nominees:

ALDI liveGfree Gluten Free Cranberry Cashew Granola

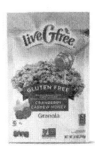

Gluten-Free Prairie Montana Mornings Granola

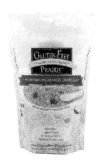

ALDI liveGfree Gluten Free Apple Almond Honey Granola

Bakery On Main's Organic Happy Granola with Sprouted Grains

ALDI liveGfree Gluten Free Raisin Almond Honey Granola

Wildway Banana Nut Gluten-free, Paleo, Grain Free Granola

Goodness Grainless Granola

Nature's Path Organic Granola Cereal, Chia Plus Coconut Chia

Best Gluten Free Ice Cream Cones

8th Annual Gluten-Free Awards:

1st Place: Let's Do Organic Ice Cream Cones, Gluten Free

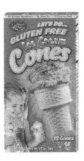

2nd Place: Goldbaum's Gluten Free Ice Cream Cone

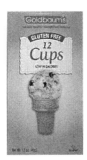

3rd Place: Edward & Sons Trading Co Cones, Sugar, Gluten Free

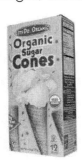

Other Nominees:

Barkat Gluten Free Waffle Ice Cream Cones

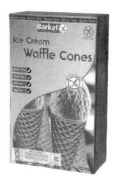

Article: On Relationships, "Celiac Disease is your problem, not mine"

by TastyMeditation

One of the questions that I get asked the most is "How did your friends and family respond to the news of your Celiac diagnosis?" When I was first diagnosed I had heard many horror stories of significant others/family members being...less than kind. I thought that my situation was pretty good – Mom was going gluten free with me; Sister was looking up the best gluten free cupcake recipe; even crazy Grandma bought me a gluten free cookbook (she bought one for herself, too – "I think I have a touch of the Celiac." Great, Grandma.....). The place where I struggled was in one particular relationship. "Jessica, what's your boyfriend like? Is he supportive?" I remember giving a lot of painful smiles. Let's call my then-boyfriend Mike.

My doctor was thrilled with my progress. I was his star patient. He marveled at my positive attitude and how seamlessly I'd integrated the gluten free diet into my lifestyle. I began baking delicious gluten free chocolate chip cookies (Mike's favorite) and compiled a list of dozens of gluten free restaurants in my city. Yet despite my many efforts to make going gluten free a positive experience, Mike always found ways to put me down.

He started complaining – said that I was never all that sick to begin with and refused to believe I could become ill from things like crumbs, shared cooking utensils, or a kiss. He complained about not being able to eat at any restaurant we happened to stumble upon. He raised his voice at me when (after he ate gluten-filled Chinese food) I kissed him on the cheek rather than on the lips. He told me that he hated my diagnosis and wanted to be able to kiss me whenever he wanted to. "This is your problem, not mine," he said.

I finally came to terms with reality. This was not going to work. No matter how many times I explained Celiac and asked for his help, he showed me that my health wasn't important to him. And this was something that I generally had control over – I had turned my life around without the need of medication or surgery. In the future, what would happen if I were diagnosed with something more serious? Would he love and support me if I got cancer? Developed Alzheimer's? My guess is no.

I am happy to now have a boyfriend who is supportive of my needs and knows that my health is a priority. Towards the end of our first date, the topic of food came up. Hesitating slightly, I told him about Celiac Disease, preparing myself for the familiar eye rolling and huffy attitude. But it didn't happen. "Oh one of my old roommates has Celiac Disease." It was a non-issue. The first time he made dinner for me at his apartment (if you ask him about it he'll blush and say that grilled cheese and soup from a carton is hardly "making dinner") he went to the store and bought a loaf of Udi's bread and a new pan/spatula to be used only for gluten free cooking (#SoThisIsLove).

Our loved ones may not fully understand the pain, confusion and stress that can be associated with

Celiac Disease, but we can and should expect acceptance and kindness. My dear grandparents always forget that you cannot wash breadcrumbs off of meat, but they care and try to understand (and they are not offended when I don't eat their chicken).

No one berates people with cancer. No one tries to convince someone who is prone to seizures that just a little bit of strobe lighting can't hurt them. No one refuses to believe that heart attacks don't exist. Why do people think it's okay to do this with Celiac sufferers? Making fun of and belittling someone's medical condition is emotionally abusive. Enabling them to forgo their treatment is wrong.

I can de-friend Mike on Facebook, but similar issues with close family members are difficult. Be vocal about your needs. Be patient with them (it's a learning process). But in the end, always put your health and safety first.

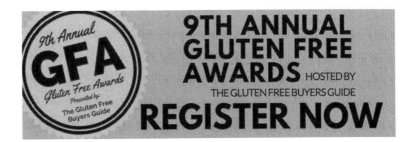

DID YOU KNOW?

GLUTEN CAN'T BE DIGESTED BY HUMAN BODY (LONG CHAIN AMINO ACID)

Quoted from:
17th International Celiac Disease
Symposium in New Delhi, India

Best Gluten Free Jerky

8th Annual Gluten-Free Awards:

1st Place: Oberto Original Beef Jerky

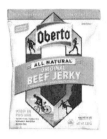

2nd Place: Krave Sweet Chipotle Beef Jerky

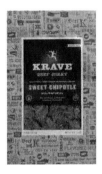

3rd Place: EPIC Bison and Bacon Bites

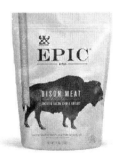

Other nominees:

Krave Pineapple Orange Beef Jerky

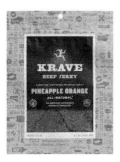

Oberto Spicy Sweet Beef Jerky

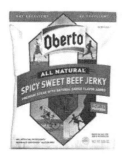

EPIC Cranberry Sriracha Beef Bites

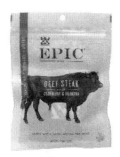

Best Gluten Free Macaroni and Cheese

8th Annual Gluten-Free Awards:

1st Place: Annie's Organic Vegan Macaroni and Cheese, Elbows & Creamy Sauce, Gluten Free Pasta

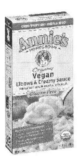

2nd Place: ALDI liveGfree Gluten Free Deluxe Macaroni & Cheese

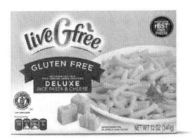

3rd Place: Daiya Mac & Cheese Cheddar Deluxe

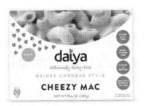

Other Nominees:

Banza Chickpea Pasta Mac & Cheese, Elbows
with White Cheddar

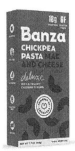

Best Gluten Free Magazines

8th Annual Gluten-Free Awards:

1st Place: Simply Gluten Free

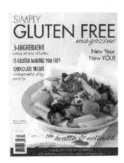

2nd Place: Living Without's Gluten Free & More

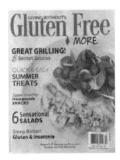

3rd Place: Gluten-Free Living

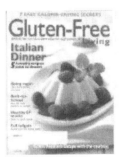

Other nominees:

Delight Gluten Free

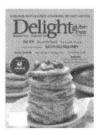

Allergic Living

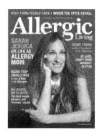

GFF Magazine

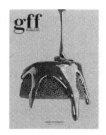

yum.

Best Gluten Free Mobile Apps

8th Annual Gluten-Free Awards:

1st Place: Find Me Gluten Free

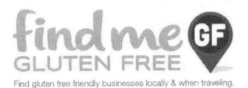

2nd Place: The Gluten Free Scanner

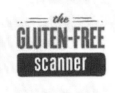

3rd Place: Epicurious

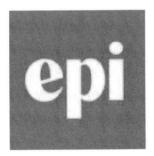

Other nominees:

ShopWell

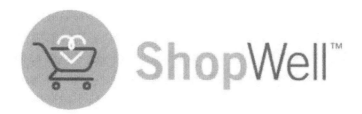

Grain or No Grain

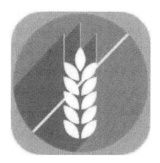

Best Gluten Free Muffin Mix

8th Annual Gluten-Free Awards:

1st Place: gfJules Muffin Mix

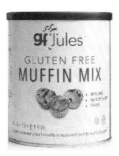

2nd Place: King Arthur Gluten Free Muffin Mix

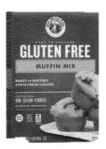

3rd Place: Bob's Red Mill Gluten Free Muffin Mix

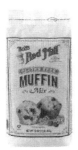

Other nominees:

Enjoy Life Muffin Mix

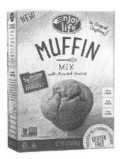

Simple Mills Gluten Free Pumpkin Muffin Mix

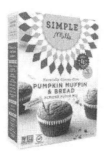

Namaste Foods, Gluten Free Muffin Mix

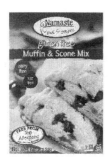

Bona Dea Ancient Grains Baking Mix Muffins

Best Gluten Free Munchies

8th Annual Gluten-Free Awards:

1st Place: LÄRABAR Bites Caramel Sea Salt

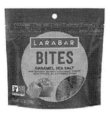

2nd Place: Three Bakers Real Cheddar Cheese Snackers

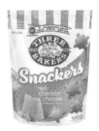

3rd Place: LÄRABAR Bites Mint Chocolate Truffle

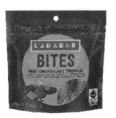

Other nominees:

Three Bakers Chocolate Chocolate Chip Snackers

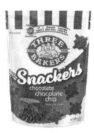

Mary's Gone Crackers - Grab 'N' Go Super Seed Classic Crackers

Earth Balance Vegan Aged White Cheddar Popcorn

Enjoy Life Foods Garlic & Parmesan Pelentils

Schär: Sch'nacks

Saffron Road Crunchy Chickpeas, Bombay Spice

Organic Living Superfoods Dark Chocolate Pineapple Chunks

Biena Chickpea Snacks, Rockin' Ranch

Le Veneziane Grissini Rosemary

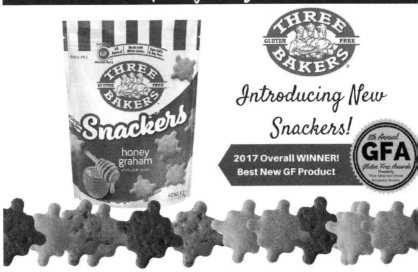
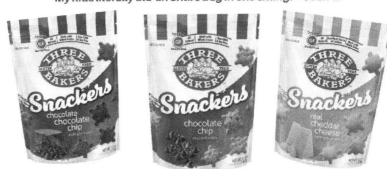

Recipe: Chocolate Vanilla Creme Cookie Truffles

by Jackie Aanonsen McEwan at Gluten Free Follow Me

Prep time

20 mins

Cook time

0 mins

Total time

20 mins

Ingredients

1 package of Glutino chocolate vanilla creme cookies

1 8oz container of whipped cream cheese

12 oz white chocolate chips

Preparation

Crush the chocolate vanilla creme cookies into fine crumbs, either in by food processor or by hand. If by hand, you can put the cookies in a resealable plastic bag and use a rolling pin.

Place 1 tbsp of cookie crumbs aside to use later.

Place the rest of the crumbs into a medium-sized bowl, and add cream cheese.

Mix the cookie crumbs and cream cheese together until well-blended.

Roll the mixture into balls, each about 1 inch diameter.

Line plate or baking sheet with parchment paper, and place cookie balls on it.

Leave the cookie balls in refrigerator for at least 30 minutes.

Melt the white chocolate chips.

Dip the cookie balls into the chocolate dip, and place on parchment paper-lined plate or baking sheet.

Sprinkle leftover cookie crumbs on each cookie truffle.

Refrigerate for at least 1 hour, or until firm.

DID YOU KNOW?

1:2 IN THE UNITED STATES WILL TRY A GLUTEN-FREE DIET THIS YEAR

Quoted from:
17th International Celiac Disease
Symposium in New Delhi, India

Best Gluten Free National Restaurant Chains

8th Annual Gluten-Free Awards:
1st Place: P.F. Chang's

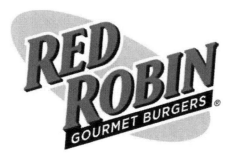

2nd Place: Red Robin

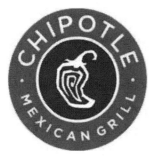

3rd Place: Chipotle

Other nominees:

Outback Steakhouse

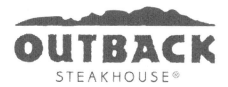

Bonefish Grill

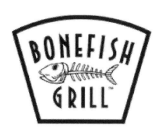

The Counter – Custom Burgers

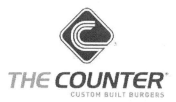

Best Gluten Free New Products

8th Annual Gluten-Free Awards:

1st Place: Enjoy Life Chocolate Chip Crunchy Mini Cookies

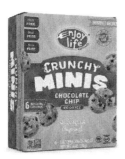

2nd Place: Schär: Artisan Baker 10 Grains and Seeds Bread

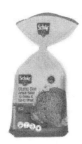

3rd Place: Enjoy Life Dark Chocolate Morsels Snack Packs

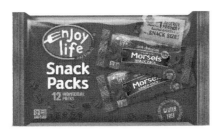

Other nominees:

Mary's Gone Crackers - Super Seed Everything

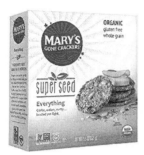

Boulder Organic Foods Chicken Noodle Soup

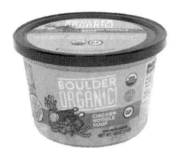

LÄRABAR Superfoods Bar Hazelnut, Hemp & Cacao

Bob's Red Mill Gluten Free Egg Replacer

Bakery On Main's Organic Creamy Hot Breakfast

Bakery On Main's Organic Happy Muesli

American Gluten Free Kids Box

Best Gluten Free Non-Profits

8th Annual Gluten-Free Awards:

1st Place: Celiac Disease Foundation (CDF)

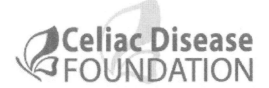

2nd Place: Gluten Intolerance Group of North America (GIG)

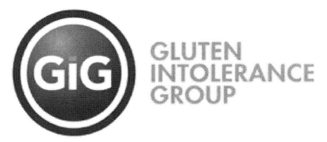

3rd Place: Beyond Celiac

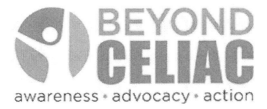

Other nominees:

Celiac Support Association (CSA) (formerly Celiac Sprue Association)

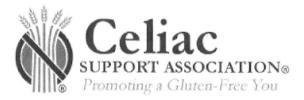

National Celiac Disease Society (NCDS)

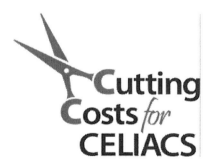

Cutting Costs for Celiacs

Best Gluten Free Online Resources

8th Annual Gluten-Free Awards:

1st Place: Celiac.org

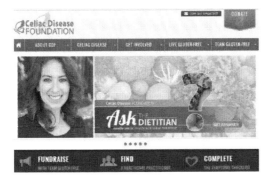

2nd Place: GlutenFreeandMore.com

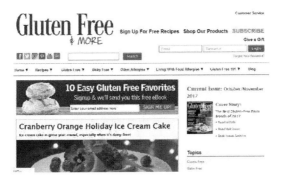

3rd Place: GlutenFreeWatchDog.org

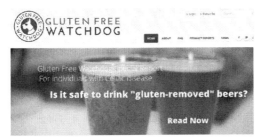

Other nominees:

Celiac.com

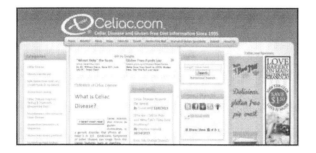

Gluten.org

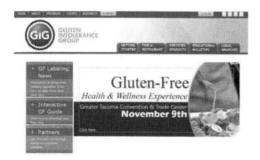

CeliacCentral.org

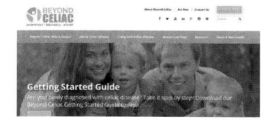

Best Gluten Free Online Stores

8th Annual Gluten-Free Awards:

1st Place: Amazon

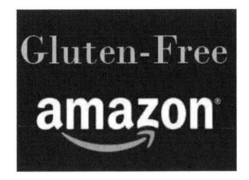

2nd Place: Gluten Free Mall

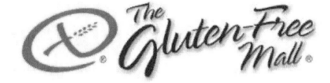

3rd Place: Thrive Market

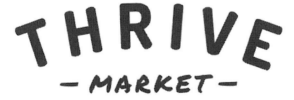

Other Nominees:

Vitacost

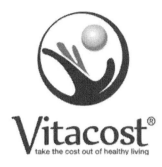

Walmart Online

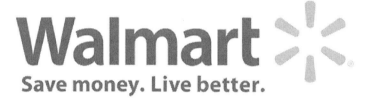

Nuts.com

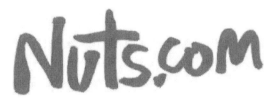

Target Online

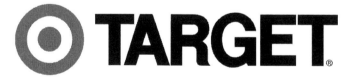

Jet.com

Best Gluten Free Pancake and Waffle Mixes

8th Annual Gluten-Free Awards:

1st Place: Pamela's Products Gluten Free Baking and Pancake Mix

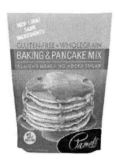

2nd Place: gfJules Pancake & Waffle Mix

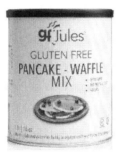

3rd Place: Enjoy Life Pancake + Waffle Mix

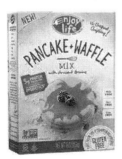

Other nominees:

Better Batter Pancake and Biscuit Mix Gluten Free

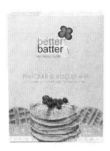

Gluten-Free Prairie Simply Our Best Pancake and Waffle Mix

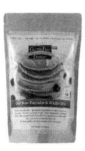

Cherrybrook Kitchen Gluten Free Pancake & Waffle Mix

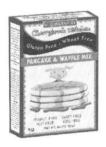

123 Gluten Free Allie's Awesome Buckwheat Pancakes

Best Gluten Free Pastas

8th Annual Gluten-Free Awards:

1st Place: Barilla

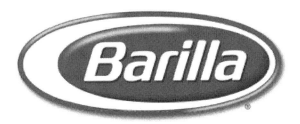

2nd Place: Tinkyada

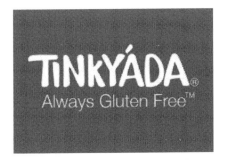

3rd Place: Ronzoni

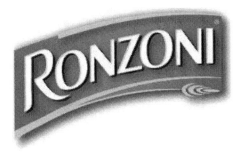

Other nominees:

Ancient Harvest Quinoa Pasta

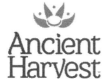

Jovial

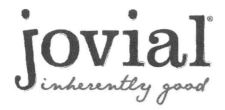

Le Veneziane Pasta

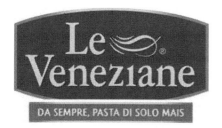

Banza

Bionature

Cappellos

Le Veneziane Potato Gnocchi

Explore Cuisine

GoGo Quinoa Super Grain

Best Gluten Free Pie Crust

8th Annual Gluten-Free Awards:

1st Place: Bobs Red Mill Gluten Free Pie Crust

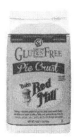

2nd Place: Glutino Perfect Pie Crust Mix

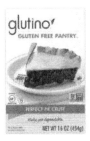

3rd Place: Gluten Free Mama, Mama's Pie Crust Mix

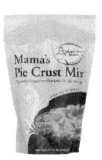

Other nominees:

The Maine Pie Co

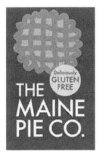

Inspiration Mix Gluten Free Pie Crust Mix

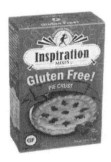

Best Gluten Free Popcorn

8th Annual Gluten-Free Awards:

1st Place: SkinnyPop

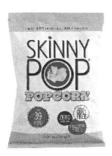

2nd Place: Smartfood

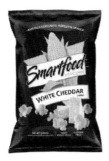

3rd Place: Bob's Red Mill White Popcorn

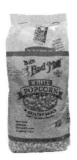

Other Nominees:

Earth Balance

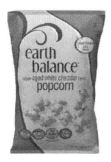

Lesser Evil

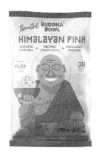

Best Gluten Free Pizza Crust

8th Annual Gluten-Free Awards:

1st Place: gfJules Pizza Crust Mix

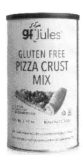

2nd Place: Bob's Red Mill Pizza Crust Mix

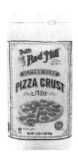

3rd Place: Three Bakers Traditional Thin Whole Grain Pizza Crust

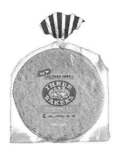

Other Nominees:

Enjoy Life Pizza Crust Mix

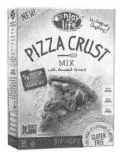

Simple Mills Pizza Dough Mix

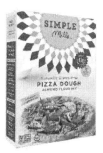

Cooqi Gluten Free Pizza & Pita Mix

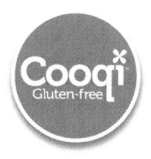

Best Gluten Free Pretzels

8th Annual Gluten-Free Awards:
1st Place: Snyder's of Hanover Gluten Free Pretzel Sticks

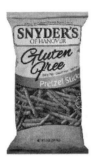

2nd Place: Glutino Pretzel Twists, Salted

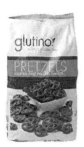

3rd Place: ALDI liveGfree Pretzel Sticks

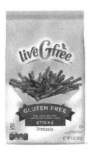

Other Nominees:

ALDI: liveGfree Pretzel Minis

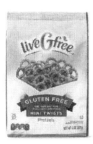

Snack Factory Gluten Free Original Pretzel Crisps

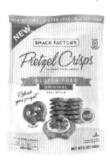

Article: Gluten Free Travel – My Top 10 Tips

by Carol Kicinski

Traveling can be one of the greatest pleasures in life and for the gluten intolerant it can also be one the most challenging. I have traveled a lot in my life, sometimes with great gluten-free success and sometimes with fairly poor results. I like to think we learn more from our failures than our successes, so here are my top 10 tips for traveling gluten-free.

1. Take food with you – Airports, train stations and roadside snack shops are not the best places to find gluten-free options. Delays at the airport can leave you famished, frustrated and more susceptible to poor decisions. Take enough gluten-free snacks (including some that contain some protein) to keep you well fed. Gluten-free pretzels or crackers, chopped fruit and vegetables, cheese cubes, gluten-free sandwiches and gluten-free nutrition bars are great items to have on hand. (At the bottom of this post is a recipe for Pistachio Fruit Bars that are delicious, easy to make, and will give you plenty of energy.)

If you take food that needs to be kept cold, put it inside a small, insulated, soft-sided lunch box and tuck in a few heavy weight Ziploc bags. After you go through security, go to a restaurant or fast food place and ask for some ice to fill the Ziplocs. This will keep everything chilled on your flight. That little lunch box will come in handy on your trip and can easily be put in your suitcase when you don't need it.

2. Plan ahead – If you are planning to travel within the United States, Triumph Dining sells this book with over 6,500 gluten-free dining options. If you don't have the book or are traveling outside the U.S., do a little research beforehand on the internet so that you arrive with some options and don't wind up starved, exhausted, and in a restaurant where you won't be able to eat anything. Of course, once you reach your destination you can do a little more digging around but it is good to arrive with a few options under your belt just in case!

3. Put it in writing – If you are traveling to a foreign country where you do not speak the language, Triumph Dining makes these cards that you can give to the server in the restaurant to ensure you get a safe, gluten-free meal. I have found that sometimes the servers don't quite get it, so if they look confused or give you a glib response, make sure you get the card to the chef. They will understand much better. If you don't have the cards, ask the concierge at your hotel to write out a simple statement that you can take with you to restaurants. Make sure they include that you can not eat wheat, oats, rye, or barley.

4. Don't cheat! – As much as I personally love to explore culture through food, sometimes you may need to forego the regional culinary specialty because of gluten. I have traveled in Italy and avoided pizza and pasta, France and went without bread and pastries, and China where I forewent a lot but I always found something delicious to eat. No one wants to be ill on vacation and for some people (like me) a little gluten triggers a craving for more. Considering the

long term effects of ingesting gluten when celiac or gluten intolerant – it is just not worth it.

5. Find what you CAN eat – With a little Google time you can usually find some local dishes that are naturally gluten-free. It is good to have an idea of some local delicacies you can enjoy, especially in a foreign country. This way you can experience local food culture and stay safe.

6. Fresh is best – No matter where you are, you can usually get some simple grilled fish with vegetables and salad (watch the dressing) and not have to worry about a gluten attack. When in doubt, stay away from soups, sauces, and anything fried.

When time allows, I make a point of always trying to find the local markets and buying some fresh fruits, cheeses, etc. to haveeon-hand in the hotel room or when out for the day. This is another way to explore the culture and if the street food is questionable, I will always have something to eat. Your little lunch box comes in handy here, too.

7. Drink plenty of bottled water – No matter how careful you are, you may accidentally ingest some gluten. Drinking plenty of water will help flush it out of your system faster. Also, it really helps with jet lag to stay hydrated.

8. Take probiotics – Buy the strongest probiotics you can find and take double the dose every day. This is good practice anyway for anyone with gluten intolerance but especially when traveling. This will help with digestive issues. (This is what I was recommended by my own doctor, but it may be different for you, so you are recommended to

seek medical guidance before beginning any new protocol.)

9. Take digestive enzymes – Many problems associated with gluten intolerance and celiac disease are digestive. Taking digestive enzymes before each meal, especially when traveling where you are not certain to get a completely gluten-free meal, will help break down the food and allow for greater absorption of nutrients. Enzymes also assist in normalizing the inflammatory responses if you eat a little gluten by mistake. Products like Glutenease are specifically formulated for breaking down the gluten proteins. But beware – taking Glutenease or other enzymes is NOT a license to eat gluten! They should be viewed as a precaution, not a cure.

10. Utilize the minibar – I don't mean drink the tiny $10 bottles of gin so you don't care if you eat gluten or not, I mean use the minibar to store your own perishable gluten-free snacks in your hotel room. Better yet, ask for a mini fridge to be brought to the room. I always ask but am not always accommodated, so the minibar stands in. I just take out the items that don't necessarily need to be in there (bottles of water, soda cans, bottles of liquor), store them right on top of or next to the minibar and let the hotel staff know I have not used them and will return them when I check out – this way I don't get charged for the items by mistake.

A note for people who will be camping and backpacking – You will, of course, have better control of the food you eat because you will be taking your own food with you. This is the good news. Tasty Bite makes a whole line of shelf-stable food that requires no refrigeration and is lightweight. As the name implies, they are very tasty and quick to prepare. They also are made with no preservatives and come in gluten-free, dairy-free, vegan and Kosher. You can pack up whole, healthy meals that can be prepared in just a few minutes. Supplement with some fresh foods if you are taking a cooler and you will be sure to eat well. Don't forget to take some gluten-free trail mix and jerky for hiking.

DID YOU KNOW?

CELIAC DISEASE CASES DOUBLE EVERY 15 YEARS IN THE UNITED STATES

Quoted from:
17th International Celiac Disease
Symposium in New Delhi, India

Best Gluten Free Ready Made Desserts

8th Annual Gluten-Free Awards:

1st Place: Julie's Organic Gluten Free Ice Cream Sandwiches

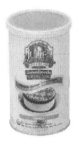

2nd Place: SO Delicious Cashew Milk Snickerdoodle Frozen Dessert

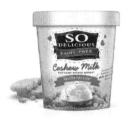

3rd Place: Katz Gluten Free, Apple Pie

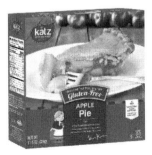

Other nominees:

Katz Gluten Free, Apple Mini Pies

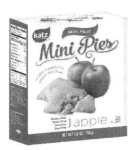

The Maine Pie Co. Single 8 Inch Gluten Free Strawberry Rhubarb Pie

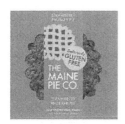

ODoughs Gluten-Free Chocolate Cake

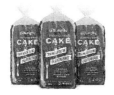

Gillian's Foods Pumpkin Gluten-Free 8 Inch Pie

The Piping Gourmets Chocolate Mint Gluten-Free Whoopie Pies

DF Mavens Mint Almond Cookie Gluten-Free Dessert Bars

Best Gluten Free Rolls

8th Annual Gluten-Free Awards:
1st Place: Schär: Ciabatta Rolls

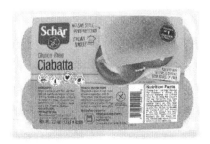

2nd Place: Three Bakers Whole Grain Hoagie Roll

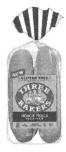 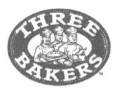

3rd Place: Bread SRSLY

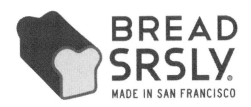

Other Nominees:

Barely Bread

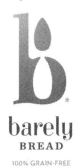

Jensen's Gluten Free Rolls

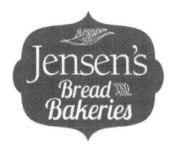

Ener-G Tapioca Dinner Rolls

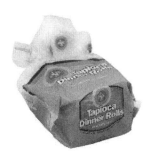

Best Gluten Free Sauces

8th Annual Gluten-Free Awards:

1st Place: San-J Organic Gluten Free Tamari Soy Sauce (Gold Label)

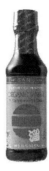

2nd Place: Kikkoman Gluten Free Soy Sauce

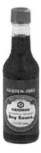

3rd Place: Organic BBQ Sauce Original

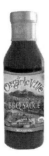

Other nominees:

Blue Top Brand Cilatro Serrano Hot Sauce

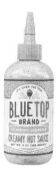

Claude's: Barbeque Brisket Marinade Sauce

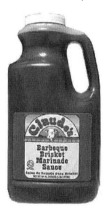

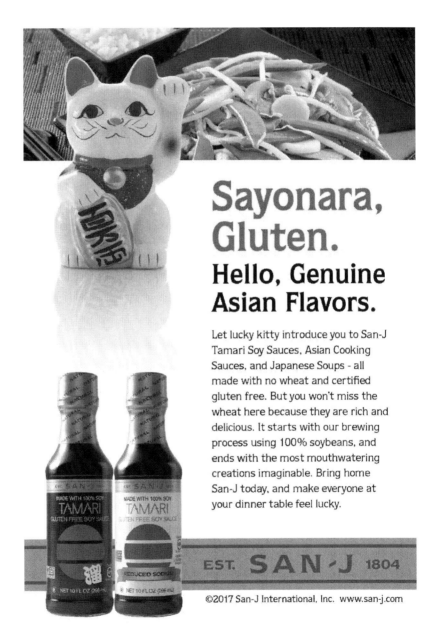

Sayonara, Gluten.

Hello, Genuine Asian Flavors.

Let lucky kitty introduce you to San-J Tamari Soy Sauces, Asian Cooking Sauces, and Japanese Soups - all made with no wheat and certified gluten free. But you won't miss the wheat here because they are rich and delicious. It starts with our brewing process using 100% soybeans, and ends with the most mouthwatering creations imaginable. Bring home San-J today, and make everyone at your dinner table feel lucky.

EST. **SAN·J** 1804

©2017 San-J International, Inc. www.san-j.com

DID YOU KNOW?

CELIAC DISEASE IS NOW AT THE CENTER-STAGE OF THE SCIENTIFIC WORLD. THE PAST DECADE HAS BEEN VERY EXCITING AND PRODUCTIVE IN TERMS OF DIAGNOSTICS AND UNDERSTANDING THE BIOLOGY OF CELIAC DISEASE. WHILE GLUTEN-FREE DIET IS THE BEST MODE OF TREATMENT, MANY OTHER TARGETS FOR CONTROL OF THE IMMUNE-PATHOGENESIS OF CELIAC DISEASE ARE NOW ACTIVELY EXPLORED, SOME OF THEM HAVE REACHED EVEN PHASE 2 AND PHASE 3 CLINICAL TRIALS.

Quoted from:
17th International Celiac Disease
Symposium in New Delhi, India

Best Gluten Free Shopping Guide

8th Annual Gluten-Free Awards:

1st Place: 2017 Gluten Free Buyers Guide by Josh and Jayme Schieffer

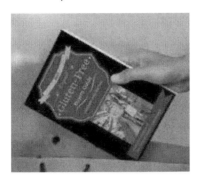

2nd Place: 2012 Essential Gluten-Free Grocery Guide Paperback – Color, April 1, 2012 by Triumph Dining Gluten Free Publishing

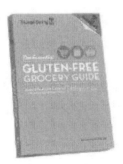

3rd Place: 2014/2015 Gluten-Free Grocery
Shopping Guide by Dr. Mara Matison, Dainis
Matison

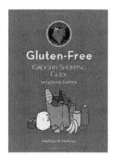

Best Gluten Free Snack Bars

8th Annual Gluten-Free Awards:
1st Place: LÄRABAR Chocolate Chip Cookie Dough

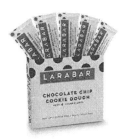

2nd Place: LUNA BAR - Gluten Free Bar - Chocolate Peppermint Stick

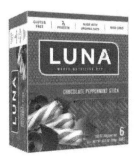

3rd Place: ALDI liveGfree Gluten Free Cocoa Loco Baked Chewy Bars

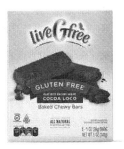

Other nominees:

LÄRABAR Peanut Butter & Jelly

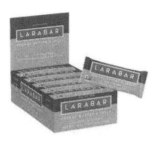

RXBAR Whole Food Protein Bar, Chocolate Sea Salt

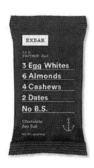

ALDI liveGfree Gluten Free Caramel Apple Baked Chewy Bars

OCHO Candy Organic Candy Bar, Peanut Butter

Enjoy Life Foods Cocoa Loco Bars

Boundless Nutrition Bar Chocolate Mint Crisp Oatmega Bar, Gluten-Free, Egg-Free

ALDI liveGfree Gluten Free Baked Very Berry Chewy Bars

Best Gluten Free Social Media Platforms

8th Annual Gluten-Free Awards:

1st Place: Facebook

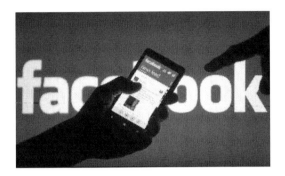

2nd Place: Pinterest

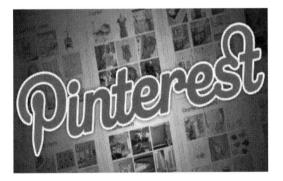

3rd Place: Instagram

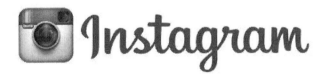

Other nominees:

Google +

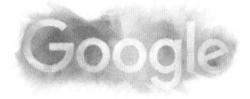

Twitter

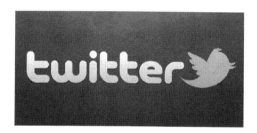

Meet-Up

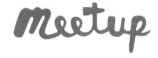

Linked In

Freedible

Best Gluten Free Soups

8th Annual Gluten-Free Awards:

1st Place: Progresso Soup Rich & Hearty New England Clam Chowder Soup Gluten Free

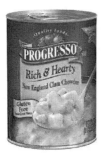

2nd Place: Gluten Free Cafe Chicken Noodle Soup

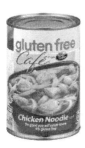

3rd Place: Amy's Organic Thai Coconut Soup (Tom Kha Phak)

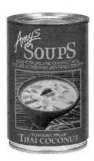

Other Nominees:

Boulder Organic Foods Roasted Tomato Basil Soup

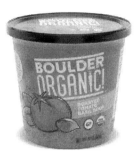

San-J White Miso Soup Envelopes

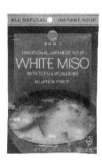

Best Gluten Free Stuffing

8th Annual Gluten-Free Awards:

1st Place: Three Bakers Herb Seasoned Stuffing Mix

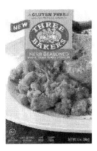

2nd Place: Aleia's Gluten Free Savory Stuffing

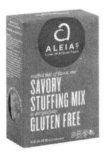

3rd Place: Gordon Rhodes - Gluten Free Sage and Onion Stuffing Mix

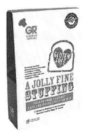

DID YOU KNOW?

AFTER BEING WELL RECOGNIZED IN EUROPE AND AMERICA, CELIAC DISEASE IS NOW GETTING RECOGNIZED IN ASIAN COUNTRIES. IT IS PREDICTED THAT THE NUMBER OF PATIENTS WITH CELIAC DISEASE IN ASIA MAY SURPASS THE NUMBERS PRESENT IN REST OF THE WORLD.

Quoted from:
17th International Celiac Disease
Symposium in New Delhi, India

Best Gluten Free Summer Camps

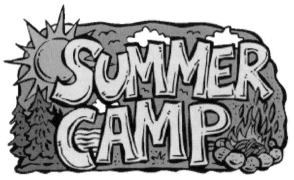

8th Annual Gluten-Free Awards:
1st Place: GIG Kids Camp WestCamp SealthVashon Island, Washington

2nd Place: Camp CeliacNorth Scituate, Rhode Island

3rd Place: Camp CeliacLivermore, California

Other Nominees:

Gluten-Free Overnight CampMiddleville, Michigan

Gluten-Free Fun CampMaple Lake, Minnesota

The Great Gluten Escape at GilmontGilmer, Texas

GIG (Gluten Intolerance Group) Kids Camp EastCamp KanataWake Forest, North Carolina

Camp WeekaneatitWarm Springs, Georgia

Camp Silly-YakBrigadoon VillageAylesford, Nova Scotia

CDF Camp Gluten-Free™ Camp Fire Camp NawakwaSan Bernardino Mountains, CA

Camp EmersonHinsdale, Massachusetts

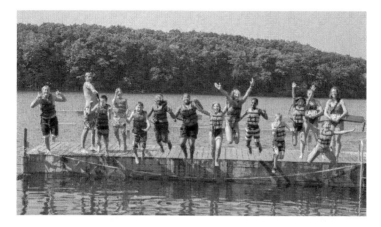

Gluten Detectives Camp (Day Camp)Bloomington, Minnesota

Appel Farm Arts CampElmer, New Jersey

International Sports Training CampPocono Mountains,Pennsylvania

Clear Creek CampGreen's Canyon, Utah (Serves Alpine School District children)

Camp TAG - Williamstown, New Jersey

Camp Eagle HillElizaville, New York

Emma Kaufmann CampMorgantown, West Virginia

Timber Lake CampShandaken, New York

Camp TAG Lebanon, Ohio at YMCA's Camp Kern.

Foundation for Children & Youth with Diabetes Camp UTADAWest Jordan, Utah

FAACT's Annual Teen Retreat

Best Gluten Free Supplements

8th Annual Gluten-Free Awards:

1st Place: Bob's Red Mill Nutritional Booster

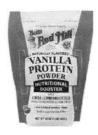

2nd Place: Vega

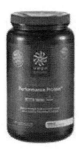

3rd Place: MegaFood

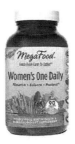

Other nominees:

Plant Fusion Protein

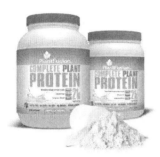

Olly

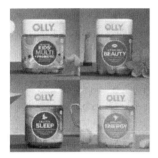

Silver Fern Ultimate Probiotic

Nuzest Protein

Growing Naturals Rice Protein

Growing Naturals Pea Protein

Best Gluten Free Tortilla or Wrap

8th Annual Gluten-Free Awards:

1st Place: Mission Soft Taco Gluten Free 8ct

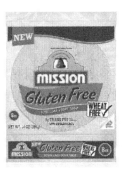

2nd Place: Rudi's Bakery Gluten Free Spinach Tortillas

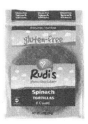

3rd Place: Toufayan Gluten Free Wraps – Original

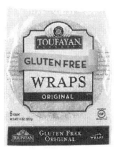

Other Nominees:

Julian Bakery Gluten Free & Keto USDA Organic Paleo Wraps

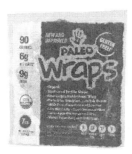

Toufayan Gluten Free Wraps – Spinach

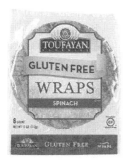

Raw Wraps Spinach- Gluten & Soy Free, Vegan & Raw, Paleo (Quinoa Seeds)

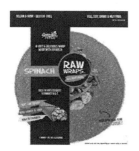

Best Gluten Free Vacation Destinations

8th Annual Gluten-Free Awards:

1st Place: Walt Disney World

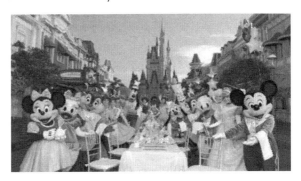

2nd Place: Italy

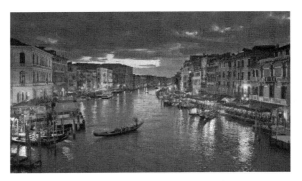

3rd Place: New York City

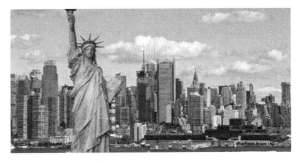

Other nominees:

Asheville, NC

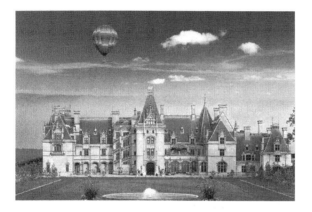

Royal Caribbean Cruises

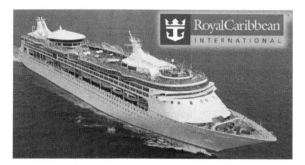

Aulani Disney Resort & Spa in Ko Olina, Hawai'i

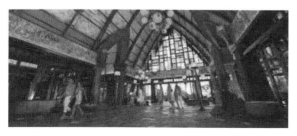

Sanara Tulum

Article: 10 Gluten-Free Kitchen Essentials for a Summer Rental

by Erin Smith

It's July 4th weekend and time to celebrate summer. Renting a beach house, cottage, lake house, or even a city-based apartment is a great alternative to a hotel on your summer vacation. I personally love to have a home away from home during a journey. I've stayed in an Airbnb in both Brooklyn and Paris. I've also rented a cottage with my family many years on Lake Erie in Canada. There is just something really comforting coming home from a long day of sightseeing or beach-ing and having a "home" and not just a hotel room.

Another perk of having a rented home is having access to a kitchen. With a kitchen, you don't have to dine out every single meal. This saves you a little bit of money and it also can help you better control what you are eating. You can buy basic essentials or you can fully stock your rental kitchen. It is really up to you and how much you want to cook during your stay. I find it super convenient to have access to a full-size fridge and basic appliances like a stove, toaster oven, and a microwave. Other travelers want someone else to take care of them during a vacation. There is no right or wrong.

Most likely, your rental kitchen is contaminated with gluten from either the owners or previous guests. Not to worry! With a few a few additions to your suitcase or carry-on bag, you can make your rental kitchen a little bit safer for your celiac-friendly vacation.

10 Gluten-Free Kitchen Essentials for a Summer Rental

Gluten-Free Food: Don't assume when you get to your summer rental that the local market will carry the same gluten-free food as your home market. Bring with you basic kitchen staples like gluten-free bread, pasta, crackers, and snacks. When you visit the local supermarket or farmer's market, look for naturally gluten-free foods like vegetables, fruits, meats, eggs, fish, and other local gluten-free delicacies.

Reusable Toaster Bags: These bags keep your toast away from crumbs in a shared toaster. They can be used in both regular toasters as well as toaster ovens for toast, grilled cheese sandwiches, or to reheat other foods that fit in the bag. The toaster bags can be washed and reused. These are a great kitchen essential!

Collapsible Bowls: The best way to keep your food from being confused with gluten-filled food is to keep it separate in completely different looking containers. These collapsible bowls not only look cool, but they pack really flat and they have covers to keep gluten crumbs from falling into your food. These can be used in a shared kitchen and are perfect for campaign too!

New Sponges: Sponges are one of those things in the kitchen that can trap gluten. Toss a few brand new sponges into your kitchen essentials bag and use those during your time using a shared kitchen. Use hot, soapy water before you even start preparing your gluten-free meal in a shared kitchen!

Roll-up Cutting Boards: Just like sponges, most cutting boards are porous and can trap gluten. There is nothing worse than preparing a meal with no gluten ingredients, only to contaminate yourself from the cutting board. These brightly-colored cutting boards lie totally flat and can be rolled up and stored away. Bonus tip: choose your "celiac" color and use that cutting board for your gluten-free food prep when you get home.

Ziploc bags: Reusable plastic bags go beyond the kitchen. Use these bags to keep open food safe from crumbs or to bring home anything that is open. You can also use these bags to store food for trips to the beach, gluten-free snacks for your bag, or even to keep your suitcase safe from open liquids on your way home. I like the gallon size the best because they hold more things.

Condiments: Some kitchens have basic staples like salt, pepper, and sugar for you to use in your rental but others are often bare. I suggest tossing a bunch of deli and restaurant condiments into a bag for you to use during the trip. This not only will help you out in a pinch (of salt, haha) but you also have "clean" condiments that have never been used before. You can also buy individual condiments like San-J Gluten-Free Tamari packets or mini bottles of Cholula hot sauce directly from Amazon.

Gluten-Free Labels: I love these little stickers! Use them at home, at school, at the office, and at your vacation rental. These labels clearly mark your food as gluten-free and hopefully keeps hungry friends and family out of your food! You can also make your own labels by using mailing address labels and a Sharpie.

Cutlery: With a good wash with soap and hot water, most cutlery should be clean from past gluten. If you want to be extra careful, I suggest bringing along some of your own cutlery. You can buy either disposable or this eco-friendly bamboo cutlery.

Foil: Use traditional aluminum foil on a shared grill or oven surface. You can lie it flat or wrap your food entirely when cooking.

Best Gluten Free Website

8th Annual Gluten-Free Awards:

1st Place: Gluten Free Watch Dog

2nd Place: Gluten Free Travel Site

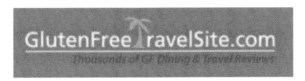

3rd Place: Cure Celiac Disease.org

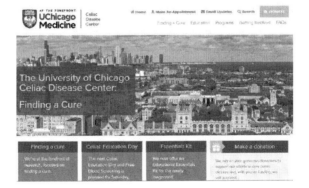

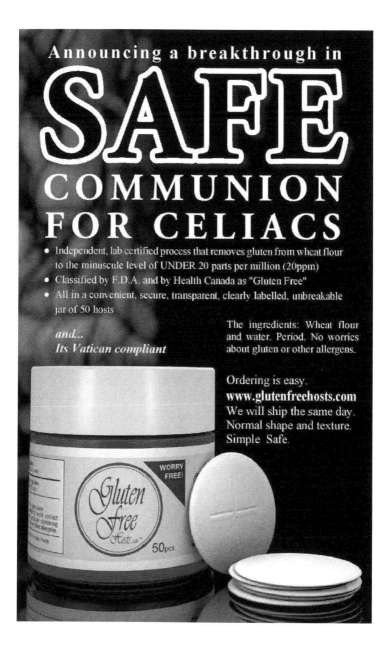

Gluten Free Product Registration

By submitting your products into The Gluten Free Awards (GFA), you are automatically entering products into the Annual Gluten Free Buyers Guide. There are only 10 slots available in each category and we limit brands to 3 submissions per category. If you are a marketer representing multiple brands, this typically will not apply. Slots can fill quickly so we recommend submitting your registration ASAP. The absolute deadline for registration is August 22nd however, we cannot guarantee you that the category is already full.

"How do I get into the Gluten Free Awards?"

How it works:
1. Fill out the registration form by adding the quantities and product names.

(A free half page ad is given for every 5 products or full-page ad for 10 products.)

2. If wanted, add additional ad space to registration.

3. Email the registration form to Jayme@GlutenFreeBuyersGuide.com

4. We will follow up with a confirmation and invoice.

If you have any questions call customer support at 828-446-1952

"Wait, I have tons of questions still"

Most common questions:

Q: I am having a hard time understanding how to submit or products.

A: Using this Registration Form will help. If lost, don't hesitate to call or email. 828-455-9734

Q: What are the image specs you need?

A: Our graphic team just needs images that are PDF, JPEG or PNG at 300 dpi or greater. The team will normally resize images based on the publishing media. Normally the product pictures and descriptions from your website will work just fine.

Q: Is there a word count for product descriptions?

A: No, we normally don't use product descriptions just product names and images.

Q: If we submit 10 products do we get 1 free full page ad and 2 free half page ads?

A: Sorry, please choose one or the other. You can always purchase additional ad space.

Q: Can we run a full page ad without entering into the awards program?

A: Yes.

Q: Do we need to send you product samples?

A: No. The gluten-free community votes for your products.

Q: Will we be in the guide if we don't win an award?

A: Yes, all products submitted will be visible as nominees.

Q: Can we use the GFA Nominee and Winner Badge on our product packaging, website and other related media?

A: Yes, we highly recommend using the badges to differentiate your products from the rest. If you happen to need higher resolution images don't hesitate to ask. Read our media terms here.

Need to talk about your order or have questions? Give us a call.

828-455-9734

or email

Josh@GlutenFreeBuyersGuide.com

From our family to yours have a happy and healthy gluten free lifestyle.

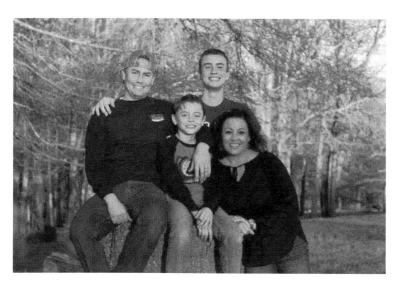

The Schieffer Family

Josh (Dad with Celiac) VP Sales and Marketing

Jayme (Mom) VP Operations

Blake (17)

Jacob (13 Celiac)

Keep up to date with us, the awards, and future buyer guides at GlutenFreeBuyersGuide.com

Made in the USA
Columbia, SC
13 December 2017